The Sad Sack Handbook

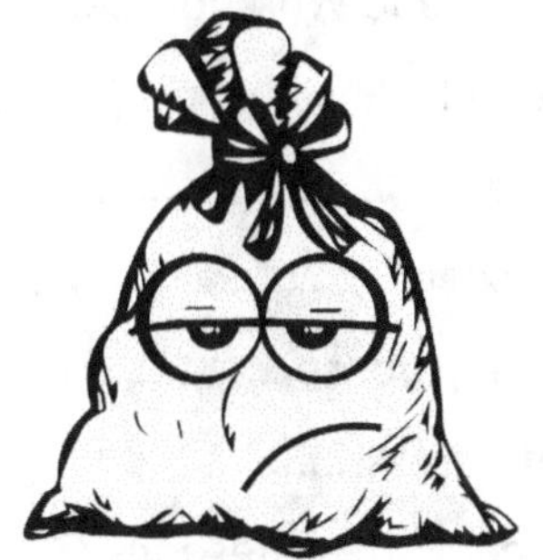

Dealing with Depression & Anxiety

By Mason Aberdeen

Table of Contents

Introduction

What is The Sad Sack Handbook?

The Sad Sack Handbook: Dealing with Depression and Anxiety is meant for people who have been coping with a depressed and uncomfortable mood. Some of the things in this guide will make more sense to younger adults, and some will make more sense to older ones. will make more sense to younger adults, and some will make more sense to older ones. Overall, this handbook tries to give an overview explanation of what depression and anxiety are and to provide practical ways to deal with them in your daily life. So, check it out for yourself. Decide which parts of this guide make sense for your life.

You might start by browsing the Table of Contents to get an idea of what topics are covered. Go over the stuff that is most interesting and pertinent to you. When you are done skimming, you can go back to the start and work through each section at your own pace. There are no right or wrong ways to use this guide and no tests! Give yourself time and be patient; you can return to sections or ideas at any time.

If you are listening to this as an audio-book, take notes or consider getting a written copy. If you are reading this on a computer, print any sections that you may want to look over again. If you have a printed copy, keep it somewhere private, so you can read it on your own time.

Throughout the handbook we've suggested things to do, write down or think about. Try to think of situations or examples that make the most sense for you. If there are ideas that don't make sense or that you are not sure about, check with someone you trust or utilize an internet search engine.

If you are nervous about other people reading what you've written, keep it private... and always remember:

If you ever get thoughts of harming yourself, tell someone you trust or if you feel like you have no one to talk to, reach out to a help line. You are never alone.

Crisis Hotline Resources

- <u>National Suicide Prevention Hotline</u> -- 1-800-273-8255

- <u>Crisis Text Line</u> -- Text Hello to 741741

- <u>YouthLine</u> -- Text teen2teen to 839863, or call 1-877-968-8491

So chin up, you sad sack, help is out there and waiting for you. Start today by not avoiding this handbook.

What is cognitive behavior therapy?

This handbook utilizes and references many ideas and techniques from cognitive behavior therapy to understand depression and anxiety. So, what is cognitive behavior therapy? And why is it important to treating depression and anxiety? Here is a brief history and explanation:

Over the past two to three decades, there has been something of a revolution in the field of psychological treatment. Sigmund Freud and his followers had a major impact on the way psychological therapy was conceptualized. Psychoanalysis and psychodynamic psychotherapy dominated the field for the first half of the 20th century. So, long-term treatments were offered, which were designed to uncover the childhood roots of personal problems, but was almost exclusively reserved for the wealthy. There was some attempt by a few health service practitioners with a public conscience to modify this form of treatment (by offering short-term treatment or group therapy), but the demand for help was so great that this had little impact. Also, while numerous case histories can be found of people who are convinced that psychotherapy did help them, practitioners of this form of therapy showed remarkably little interest in demonstrating that what they were offering their patients was, in fact, helpful.

As a reaction to the exclusivity of psychodynamic therapies and the slender evidence for its usefulness, in the 1950s and 1960s, a set of techniques were developed, broadly termed 'behavior therapy.' These techniques shared two basic features. First, they aimed to remove symptoms (such as anxiety) by dealing with those symptoms themselves, rather than their deep-seated underlying historical causes. Second, they were techniques loosely related to what laboratory psychologists were finding out about the mechanisms of learning, which were formulated in testable terms. Indeed, practitioners of behavior therapy were committed to using techniques of proven value or, at worst, of a form that could potentially be put to the test. The area where these techniques proved of most value was in the treatment of anxiety disorders, especially specific phobias (such as fear of animals or heights) and agoraphobia, both notoriously difficult to treat using conventional psychotherapies.

After an initial flush of enthusiasm, discontent with behavior therapy grew. There were a number of reasons for this, an important one of which was the fact that behavior therapy did not deal with the internal thoughts which were so obviously central to the distress that patients were experiencing. In this context, the fact that behavior therapy proved so inadequate when it came to the treatment of depression highlighted the need for major revision.

In the late 1960s and early 1970s, a treatment was developed specifically for depression called 'cognitive therapy.' The pioneer in this enterprise was an American psychiatrist, Professor Aaron T. Beck, who developed a theory of depression that emphasized the importance of people's depressed styles of thinking. He also specified a new form of therapy. Prof. Beck's work has changed the nature of psychotherapy, not just for depression but for a range of psychological problems.

In recent years, the cognitive techniques introduced by Beck have been merged with the techniques developed earlier by the behavior therapists to produce a body of theory and practice which has come to be known as 'cognitive behavior therapy.'

There are two main reasons why this form of treatment has come to be so important within the field of psychotherapy. First, cognitive therapy for depression, as originally described by Beck and developed by his successors, has been subjected to the strictest scientific testing; and it has been found to be a highly successful treatment for a significant proportion of cases of depression. Not only has it proved to be as effective as the best alternative treatments (except in the most severe cases, where medication is required), but some studies suggest that people treated successfully with cognitive behavior therapy are less likely to experience a later recurrence of their depression than people treated successfully with other forms of therapy (such as antidepressant medication). Second, it has become clear that specific patterns of thinking are associated with a range of psychological problems and that treatments that deal with these styles of thinking are highly effective. So, specific cognitive-behavioral treatments have been developed for anxiety disorders, like panic disorder, generalized anxiety disorder, specific phobias and social phobia, obsessive-compulsive disorders, and hypochondriasis (health anxiety), as well as for other conditions such as compulsive gambling, alcohol and drug addiction, and eating disorders like bulimia nervosa and binge-eating disorder.

Indeed, cognitive-behavioral techniques have a wide application beyond the narrow categories of psychological disorders: they have been applied effectively, for example, to helping people with low self-esteem and those with marital difficulties.

At any one time, almost 10 percent of the general population is suffering from depression, and more than 10 percent have one or more of the anxiety disorders. Many others have a range of psychological problems and other personal difficulties. It is important that treatments with proven effectiveness are developed and utilized. However, there remains a very great problem – namely that the delivery of treatment is expensive and the professional resources are not going to be available to everyone. While this shortfall could be met by lots of people helping themselves, commonly, the natural inclination to make oneself feel better in the present is to do precisely those things which perpetuate or even exacerbate one's problems. For example, the person with agoraphobia will stay at home to prevent the possibility of an anxiety attack; and the person with bulimia nervosa will avoid eating all potentially fattening foods. While such strategies might resolve some immediate crisis, they leave the underlying problem intact and provide no real help in dealing with future difficulties.

CBT Manuals and Workbooks

So, there is a twin problem here: although effective treatments have been developed, they are not widely available; and when people try to help themselves, they often make matters worse. In recent years the community of cognitive behavior therapists has responded to this situation. What they have done is to take the principles and techniques of specific cognitive behavior therapies for particular problems and represent them in self-help manuals and workbooks. These manuals and workbooks specify a systematic program of treatment which the individual sufferer is advised to work through to overcome their difficulties and often provide written exercises. In this way, the cognitive behavioral therapy techniques of proven value are being made available on the widest possible basis.

Although a useful tool, self-help manuals are never going to replace meeting with a therapist. Many people will need individual treatment from a qualified therapist. It is also the case that, despite the widespread success of cognitive-behavioral therapy, some people will not respond to it and will need one of the other treatments available. Nevertheless, although research on the use of cognitive-behavioral self-help manuals is at an early stage, the work done to date indicates that for a very great many people, such a manual or workbook will prove beneficial for them to identify and overcome their problems.

Many people suffer silently and secretly for years. Sometimes appropriate help is not forthcoming despite their efforts to find it. Sometimes they feel too ashamed or guilty to reveal their problems to anyone. For many of these people, the cognitive-behavioral self-help manuals and workbooks will provide a lifeline to recovery and a better future. While this guide provides some useful exercises, you can find many more examples in manuals and workbooks online or through your local book retailer. Try searching for terms like 'cbt', 'cbt manual' or 'cbt work-book.'

Introduction to Anxiety and Depression:

Depression and anxiety can occur at the same time. In fact, it's been estimated that 45 percent of people with one mental health condition meet the criteria for two or more disorders. But depressed people do get better, and depression does end. There are effective treatments and self-help skills to deal with depression. Health care professionals give depression treatments, but you can learn self-help skills and apply them to your own life. This guide teaches a set of antidepressant skills you can use to overcome depression. Sometimes the skills can be used on their own when the depression isn't too severe. Sometimes they have to be used along with treatments by professionals.

While anxiety and depression are different conditions, they share many causes and some symptoms. This can sometimes lead people to think they have, for example, depression, when they're actually experiencing an anxiety condition. It is not uncommon for anxiety and depression to occur together – over half of those who experience depression also experience symptoms of an anxiety condition – and in some cases, one can lead to the onset of the other.

The good news is that, just like physical conditions, anxiety and depression can be treated. Both conditions share many of the same treatments, and with the right treatment, people can recover. The sooner a person with anxiety and/or depression seeks support, the sooner he or she can recover. This book aims to provide clear and comprehensive information about anxiety and depression, including:

- What the conditions are

- Common symptoms and how to recognize them

- How to get support for yourself or for someone you know

- How to stay well.

Part 1: Anxiety

What is Anxiety?

Anxiety is an emotion characterized by feelings of tension, worried thoughts, and physical changes like increased blood pressure. While anxiety can cause distress, it is not always a medical condition. Anxiety is a normal or often healthy emotion. When an individual faces potentially harmful or worrying triggers, feelings of anxiety are not only normal but necessary for survival.

Everyone feels anxiety from time to time. Most people experience anxiety at some point in their lives. Anxiety is the emotion we feel when we think we are under threat and cannot cope with a situation. Common situations that might make people feel anxious are exams, job interviews, or public speaking. Anxiety is an emotion experienced by everyone. But for some people, anxiety can seem unbearable. It can feel like anxiety is always there. Indeed, it can be experienced so intensely that it stops people from doing what they want to do in life. Therefore, anxiety can be very distressing. Few people get through a week without some anxious tension or a feeling that something is not going to go well.

We may feel anxiety when we're facing an important event, such as an exam or job interview, or when we perceive some threat or danger, such as waking to strange sounds in the night. However, such everyday anxiety is generally occasional, mild, and brief, while the anxiety felt by the person with an anxiety disorder occurs frequently, is more intense, and lasts longer—up to hours, or even days. Unfortunately, anxiety disorders are common. Research shows that up to one in four adults has an anxiety disorder sometime in their life and that one person in 10 is likely to have had an anxiety disorder in the past year.

Anxiety disorders are the most common mental health problem in women and are second only to substance use disorders in men. Anxiety disorders can make it hard for people to work or study, to manage daily tasks, and to relate well with others, and often result in financial strain and profound personal suffering. People often live with anxiety disorders for years before they are diagnosed and treated. If you suspect that you have an anxiety disorder, it is important to seek professional treatment as soon as possible. Anxiety disorders are treatable, and early treatment can help to ensure treatment success.

Normal-Anxiety

Worries, fear, and anxieties are common to us all. They are the normal reactions to stress or danger and only become a problem when they are exaggerated or experienced out of context.

Normal-Anxiety is a normal experience, which, although unpleasant, is harmless. Some examples of anxiety symptoms are:

feeling nervous or on edge, an increased heart rate, shortness of breath, a dry mouth, trembling, sweating, nausea, light-headedness, and thinking that something bad is going to happen. This is not an exhaustive list, and there are many other common symptoms of anxiety. Although unpleasant, anxiety can actually be very helpful. In fact, it can warn and protect us when we are in danger.

A certain amount of anxiety is normal and necessary; it can lead you to act on your concerns and protect you from harm. In some situations, anxiety can even be essential to your survival. If you were standing at the edge of a curb, for example, and a car swerved toward you, you would immediately perceive danger, feel alarmed and jump back to avoid the car. Most of us would feel anxious standing on the edge of a cliff without any barriers. The feeling of anxiety motivates us to move away from the edge or be very careful if remaining on edge. Therefore, anxiety alerts us to possible danger and prepares our body to respond to the danger.

Since the earliest days of humanity, the approach of predators and incoming danger sets off alarms in the body and allows evasive action. These alarms become noticeable in the form of a raised heartbeat, sweating, and increased sensitivity to surroundings. The danger causes a rush of adrenalin, a hormone and chemical messenger in the brain, which in turn triggers these anxious reactions in a process called the "fight-or-flight" response.

This prepares humans to physically confront or flee any potential threats to safety. For many people, running from larger animals and imminent danger is a less pressing concern than it would have been for early humans. Anxieties now revolve around work, money, family life, health, and other crucial issues that demand a persons' attention without necessarily requiring the fight-or-flight reaction. The nervous feeling before an important life event or during a difficult situation is a natural echo of the original 'fight-or-flight' reaction. It can still be essential to survival – anxiety about being hit by a car when crossing the street, for example, means that a person will instinctively look both ways to avoid danger. Anxiety is your body's natural response to stress. Its' a feeling of fear or apprehension about whats' to come. The first day of School, going to a job interview, or giving a speech may cause most people to feel fearful and nervous.

When we feel danger or think that danger is about to occur, the brain sends a message to the nervous system, which responds by releasing adrenaline. Increased adrenaline causes us to feel alert and energetic and gives us a spurt of strength, preparing us to attack (fight) or escape to safety (flight). Increased adrenaline can also have unpleasant side-effects. These can include feeling nervous, tense, dizzy, sweaty, shaky, or breathless. Such effects can be disturbing, but they are not harmful to the body and generally do not last long.

The fight-or-flight response

The fight-or-flight response has evolved over millions of years to enable us to confront or escape danger. This response includes:

- Breathing more quickly to get more oxygen to the muscles

- Increased heart rate to increase blood flow to the muscles

- Increased muscle tension to be able to react quickly

- Digestion slows down

- Saliva production decreases, causing a dry mouth

- A release of adrenaline, which can cause trembling

- Sweating to cool the body down in anticipation of physical exertion

- The mind becomes focused on the threat or scans our environment for further threat

When the danger has passed, the body returns to a less anxious state.

Anxiety is more than just feeling stressed or worried. While stress and anxious feelings are a common response to a situation where a person feels under pressure, it usually passes once the stressful situation has passed, or 'stressor' is removed.

Anxiety is when these anxious feelings don't subside. Anxiety is when they are ongoing and exist without any particular reason or cause. It's a serious condition that makes it hard for a person to cope with daily life. We all feel anxious from time to time, but for a person experiencing anxiety, these feelings cannot be controlled.

Now, let us take a more in depth look at our natural reactions to situations and their relationship, good and bad, to anxiety by examining an example of the "Stress Response."

The Stress Response

"It couldn't have been more idyllic. A peaceful summer's day in the country, just me and my young son. Then I heard the rattle and saw that it was slithering towards us. I felt a whoosh of adrenaline, and my heart jumped into my throat. The hair on the back of my neck bristled, my body tensed, and all I could think of was my son's safety. I had to get him to safety. I scooped him up and ran. I forgot his toys; I forgot the camera, I was so focused on the gate at the edge of the field and our escape. I don't know where the energy came from, but I found the strength to carry him, and I was able to get to the gate before the snake reached us. Afterward, I felt jittery and exhausted, but this eased off with time."

Worry, fear, and anxiety are crucial to our survival because they prepare us for coping with stress or danger. They trigger the release of a hormone (adrenaline), which promotes physical and mental changes that prepare us for either taking on a challenge or fleeing from a dangerous situation. Once the stress or danger has passed, these temporary changes subside. Our ancestors were faced with very tangible threats to their safety, such as a wild animal or a hostile neighbor, so for them, this fight-flight response was highly appropriate. The stresses which we face today tend to be more subtle: delays, ongoing domestic problems, deadlines, job loss. Nonetheless, we experience the same bodily, mental, and behavioral changes as did our ancestors.

The Bodily Changes

. . . I felt a whoosh of adrenaline, and my heart jumped into my throat. The hair on the back of my neck bristled, my body tensed . . .

The bodily responses that we are likely to experience include heightened muscular tension, increased breathing rate, raised blood pressure, perspiration and digestive changes.

All of these reactions increase our readiness for action and explain many of the bodily sensations that we associate with anxiety, such as tense muscles, panting, racing heart, sweating, 'butterflies.' This is the ideal state for someone who has to react with a burst of energy: the athlete who is about to run an important race, for example. Without these physical changes, he would be sluggish rather than primed for action.

The Psychological Changes

. . . all I could think of was my son's safety. I had to get him to safety. I scooped him up and ran. I forgot his toys; I forgot the camera, I was so focused on the gate at the edge of the field and our escape . . .

The psychological changes associated with stress include changes in the way we think and sometimes in the way we feel, which, again, help us to cope under stress. When faced with danger or stress, our thinking becomes more focused, and there can be an improvement in concentration and problem-solving. This is an ideal state of mind for anyone facing a serious challenge – a surgeon carrying out an operation, a stockbroker making a swift decision about an investment, a parent restraining a child who is about to walk into the road. Without the stress response, their reactions might be too careless. We can also experience a range of emotional responses to stress, such as increased irritability or even a sense of well-being. Imagine the stressed father becoming short-tempered with his children or the executive who becomes exhilarated as she gets closer to meeting her stressful deadlines, or the excited teenager watching a horror film.

The Behavioral Changes

. . . I don't know where the energy came from, but I found the strength to carry him, and I was able to get to the gate before the bull reached us . . .

The behavioral responses to stress or danger are usually forms of escape or vigilance (i.e., flight or fight). If I see a tree branch falling towards me, I get a burst of energy and jump out of the way in order to escape. If I am driving and go into a skid, I become particularly determined to correct this, and I find the strength to hold on to the steering wheel. Again, these are vital reactions: without such changes in behavior, I would find myself trapped under a branch or caught up in an uncontrolled skid. Thus, the bodily, mental, and behavioral responses to stress are normal, helpful, and often vital, and, up to a point, our ability to cope with stress improves as we undergo more stress. This is shown in the stress-and-performance graph which shows a correlation between increased stress level and increased performance. At the bottom of the curve, when performance and stress level are at their lowest, we are relaxed but physically and mentally ill-equipped to deal with danger because we are not primed for action when we are in this state. As our stress level rises, our body and mind become increasingly able to confront stress.

Long-Term Stress

"I used to be positive about myself and had energy and ideas, but I've lost all that since we started to go through a crisis with the business. Now I really have to push myself to do routine things because I feel so tired and dull. Even when I do get things done, I get no enjoyment from it, and so every-thing feels like a chore. It doesn't end there because I go home worrying about the business and about my performance. I can't get these things out of my mind, so I don't even bother to try to be sociable anymore. Sometimes I feel quite ill with it all, and I haven't slept properly in months. I can't understand how I can push myself and not seem to get anywhere."

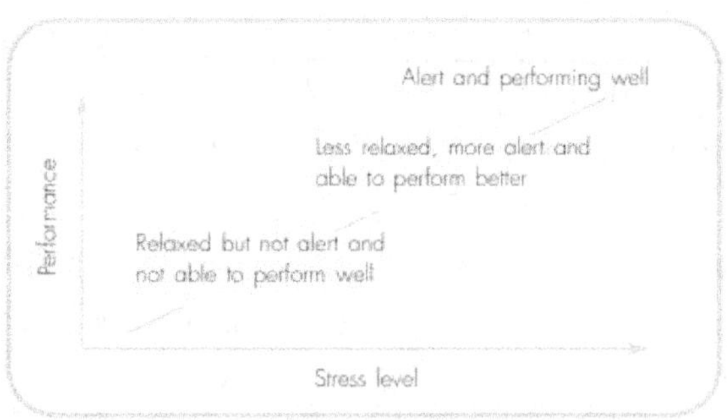

Clearly, the changes brought about in the stress response are helpful in the short term because they prepare our bodies for physical activity and focus our minds on the immediate problem. However, they evolved as an immediate and temporary response to stress, which was switched off as soon as the danger passed. Problems can arise if these reactions are not switched off, that is, if the stress response becomes chronic or excessive. If this happens, we pass our peak, and per-formance begins to deteriorate:

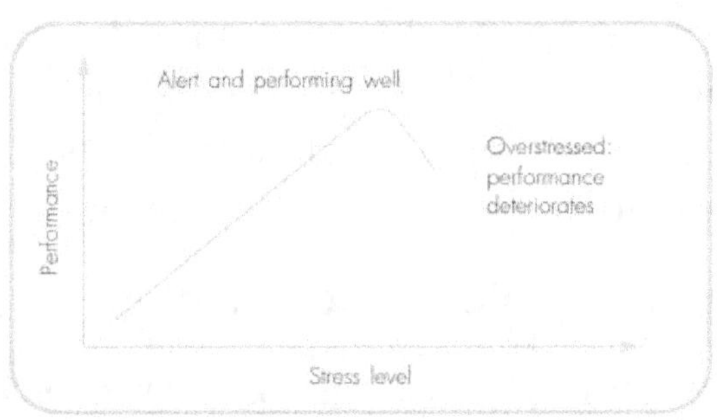

The Bodily Changes

The bodily sensations now become more unpleasant. The muscular tension, so important for fight and flight, can develop into muscular discomfort throughout the body. This might be experienced as headaches; difficulty in swallowing; shoulder, neck, and chest pain; stomach cramps; trembling, and weak legs.

With prolonged or extreme stress, a person can become aware of the heart-pounding and, as blood pressure rises, begin to experience light-headedness, blurred vision, ringing in the ears. As the breathing rate increases, one might feel dizzy, nauseous, and short of breath. If the digestive system is affected by prolonged stress, sickness, diarrhea, and stomach pain can result. Finally, sweating can become excessive and, although this is not harmful, it can cause embarrassment.

The Psychological changes

The psychological reactions, if sustained, cause thinking to become far too focused on worrying so that a person always fears the worst, worrying that a problem is impossible to solve and generally thinking negatively. Such negative thinking can form a vicious cycle with the bodily changes during stress if physiological reactions trigger worries such as: '*Pains in my chest. There's something wrong with my heart!*' or '*This feeling is unbearable, and there's nothing I can do about it.*' This will keep stress levels high and prolong the physical discomfort and, therefore, the worrying.

The emotional changes which can occur because of ongoing worry and anxiety are typically those of irritability, constant fearfulness, and demoralization. When any of us is feeling like this, we find it much more difficult to cope with stress, and when our coping resources are low, the stress is much more likely to get on top of us.

The Behavioral Changes

The changes in behavior, if persistent, can also give rise to difficulties. Constant fidgeting and rushing around becomes exhausting, making one tired and less able to handle stress. Increased comfort eating, smoking, or drinking can cause physical and mental problems and take a toll on one's health and sense of well-being. The most common response to fear is running away or avoiding the situation or object which triggers fear. However, the relief obtained from avoidance is often only temporary and leads to a loss of self-confidence so that the situation soon becomes even more difficult to face.

You can see that the response to stress can itself become distressing. This might be because the physical changes are alarming, or because the worrying and the emotional changes impair one's ability to cope, or because a loss of self-confidence makes it difficult to face fears and overcome them. Whatever the reason, when the natural stress response causes more distress, a cycle has been created, which is difficult to contro. This cycle, which maintains the stress response after it has been triggered, is the common factor in all forms of problem worry, fear, and anxiety.

What Triggers Stress Response?

The actual trigger for the stress response might be any real or imagined threat. For example, a man with a snake phobia would experience distress on seeing a real snake or on coming across a picture of a snake. He would have the same response if he believed that he had seen a snake or if he believed that he was likely to come into contact with a snake in a zoo, for example. A woman who was fearful of public speaking would feel panicky as she stood to give a speech at a wedding, but she might feel just as afraid if she believed that she would be asked to stand up and speak without warning.

Do I Have Anxiety?

The symptoms of anxiety can often develop over time gradually. Given that we all experience some anxiety, it can be hard to know how much is too much. In order to be diagnosed with an anxiety condition, it must have a disabling impact on the person's life.

There are many types of anxiety, and there is a range of symptoms for each. Some common symptoms include:

- hot and cold flushes
- racing heart
- tightening of the chest
- snowballing worries
- obsessive thinking
- compulsive behavior.

If you are familiar with any of these symptoms, check the more extensive list of symptoms below.

Common Symptoms of Anxiety

Behavior

- Withdrawing from, avoiding, or enduring with fear objects or situations that cause anxiety

- Urges to perform certain rituals to try and relieve anxiety

- Not being assertive (i.e., avoiding eye contact)

- Difficulty making decisions

- Being startled easily

Physical

- Increased heart rate/racing heart

- Shortness of breath

- Vomiting, nausea, or stomach pain

- Muscle tension and pain (e.g., sore back or jaw)

- Feeling detached from your physical self or surroundings.

- Having trouble sleeping (e.g., difficulty falling or staying asleep)

- Sweating, shaking

- Dizzy, lightheaded or faint

- Numbness or tingling

- Hot or cold flushes

- Difficulty concentrating

Thoughts

- "I am going crazy."

- "I can't control myself."

- "I'm about to die."

- "People are judging me."

- Having upsetting dreams or flashbacks of a traumatic event

- Finding it hard to stop worrying

- Unwanted or intrusive thoughts

Feelings

- Overwhelmed

- Fear (particularly when having to face certain objects, situations, or events)

- Worried about physical symptoms (e.g., fearing there is an undiagnosed medical problem)

- Dread (e.g., that something bad is going to happen)

- Constantly tense, nervous, or feeling on the edge

- Uncontrollable or overwhelming panic

The list of symptoms is not designed to provide a diagnosis – for that, you need to see a doctor – but it can be used as a guide.

What Causes Anxiety?

A combination of factors lead to a person developing anxiety, including the following:

Life Events: Often, we develop anxiety following a series of stressful life events. This is especially true if we experience many different pressures all at once. For example, if someone has work pressures, financial difficulties, and relationship problems, all at the same time, it is perhaps unsurprising that they become anxious. When thinking about it in this way, anxiety is often the result of feeling as though we cannot cope with the demands placed upon us. In addition, people can learn to be anxious based on their life experiences. For example, if someone has faced workplace bullying in the past, they may be more likely to suffer anxiety when beginning a new job.

Thinking Styles: Some people may have a thinking style that lends itself to experiencing anxiety. For example, anxious people have a tendency to expect that the worst possible scenario will always occur. They also feel like they must constantly be on guard in case something bad happens. They believe that by thinking about all the things that could go wrong, they will be better prepared to cope if it happens. However, thinking in these ways means they are on regular alert and find it difficult to relax and 'switch off.'

Evolutionary Reasons: We also experience anxiety because of its evolutionary benefits. Put another way, although anxiety is largely an unpleasant experience, it also has positive benefits that have been useful to humans over the centuries. For example, when we are under threat or feel in danger (e.g., hear a burglar), we automatically become anxious. As a result, our heartbeats more quickly, which supplies blood to our muscles (which helps us run away from or fight the burglar); we sweat (which cools us down during this process); and our breathing changes (which ensures oxygen is delivered to our muscles quickly, again preparing us for a quick response). When looking at anxiety in this way, you can quickly see how it can be very useful in certain situations.

Biological Reasons: It has also been suggested that anxiety has familial ties. In other words, if someone in your immediate family is an anxious person, there is an increased chance that you will have similar personality traits.

In reality, it is likely that a combination of all these factors influences someone's anxiety levels. However, in some ways, it is less important to know what causes anxiety and more important to know what stops us from overcoming it.

What Keeps Our Anxiety Going?

Some people have a style of thinking which lends itself to experiencing anxiety. For example, it appears that some people are more likely to overestimate the likelihood of bad things happening than others. It is easy to see how regularly presuming the worst in this way would make someone feel anxious. Unfortunately, when we do feel anxious, we become even less likely to think as clearly as we would like, and a vicious cycle occurs.

Anxious people also sometimes believe that worrying has a protective function. More specifically, they believe that being on the 'lookout' for danger can help them to recognize and avoid it. Unfortunately, when searching for danger in this way, they soon begin seeing potential danger in many relatively safe situations, which of course, makes them feel anxious. They may also believe that by considering everything that could go wrong, they will be better prepared to cope when it does. However, often these beliefs mean a lot of extra time is spent worrying than is necessary, as many of our worries never come true. Of course, the more time we spend worrying, the more anxious we feel.

Another way someone's thinking style can keep their anxiety going is because they become 'worried about worrying.' Here, people tend to worry that they are doing harm to themselves (e.g., going mad) by worrying so often (which is not the case), and a vicious cycle occurs. Similarly, people often worry about the physical symptoms they experience when they are anxious (e.g., breathlessness, rapid heart rate, etc.). Unfortunately, worrying about these symptoms (which are perfectly safe and natural bodily reactions) only makes them feel worse, again creating a vicious cycle of anxiety.

One other important factor that can keep people's anxiety going is that they often change their behavior as a result of their anxiety. For example, they may avoid going to a party because they have spotted many potential 'dangers' (e.g., "what if no one likes me"). Similarly, they may put off completing an assignment because they worry about it being negatively evaluated. Unfortunately, because people tend to use such avoidance strategies, they can never see that things would often go better than they thought, and their anxiety remains as a result.

Not having enough free time to relax and do the things we enjoy can also contribute to our higher anxiety levels. On the other hand, having too much free time can mean we have lots of opportunities to engage in worry and feel anxious.

How can I reduce anxiety?

Fortunately, there are a number of strategies that we can use to reduce our anxiety. These include:

1. Understanding more about anxiety.

2. Learning how to challenge your unhelpful thoughts and see things in a more realistic light.

3. Improving problem-solving skills.

4. Learning how to reduce the amount of time you spend worrying.

5. Learning how you can feel more relaxed (Physically and mentally).

6. Learning how to stop avoiding the things that make you anxious.

When going through this book, it can sometimes be more helpful to try out the ideas above one at a time, rather than trying to learn them all at once. However, simply take your own pace.

Understanding Anxiety

Anxiety is undoubtedly an unpleasant feeling, but it is something that everyone experiences. Of course, some people experience anxiety more regularly than others, but it is a completely natural experience that is part and parcel of daily life. Due to the unpleasant nature of anxiety, people often worry that experiencing it is harmful. For example, they may fear that regularly worrying will make them go mad or that the physical symptoms of anxiety (e.g., heart racing) are signs of a serious health problem. Such fears naturally make people even more anxious, which creates a vicious cycle of anxiety.

However, when exploring anxiety more closely, we can see that it is a very healthy response which actually helps to protect us. By learning more about anxiety and why we experience it in the first place, we can see that it is not harmful. This can help us to be less fearful of the symptoms, which in turn has a positive effect on our overall anxiety levels.

As mentioned earlier, the symptoms we experience when anxious are often referred to as the 'fight or flight' response. This comes from the idea that people primarily experience anxiety to help them either fight or run away from danger. For example, if you saw a burglar, two options open to you would be to either - fight them off (fight) or try to run away (flight). Our fight or flight response would kick in to help us at this point. For example:

- Our hearts would begin beating more quickly (supplying blood to our muscles).

- We would sweat (to cool us down).

- Our muscles would become tense (ready for action).

- We would take deeper breaths (to supply oxygen to our muscles).

In essence, all of these responses would aid our escape or improve our ability to stay and fight the intruder. When considered in this way, we can see how the symptoms of anxiety are helpful to us. Indeed, all of the physical symptoms we experience when anxious play a helpful role in protecting us in such circumstances.

This fight or flight response was likely even more vital to human survival back in the days of early man when people had to hunt for their food and were under a greater threat from predators. Nowadays, we do not face the same threats, but unfortunately, our bodies and minds have not caught up with these changes. As a result, we now experience anxiety in situations where it is not necessarily as helpful because we cannot fight or run away from them (e.g., work or financial pressures). However, the one thing that has stayed true is the fact that these symptoms are not dangerous; it is in many ways the right response but at the wrong time. Remembering this can help you to be less fearful of the symptoms of anxiety, which will allow them to pass sooner.

Challenging Unhelpful Thoughts

The way that we think about things has an impact on our anxiety levels. Many of these thoughts occur outside of our control and can be negative or unhelpful. It is therefore important to remember that they are just thoughts, without any real basis, and are not necessarily facts. Even though we may believe a lot of our unhelpful thoughts when we are anxious, it is good to remember that they should be questioned as they are often based on wrong assumptions.

The following section will help you begin to recognize if you are thinking about things in an unhelpful or unrealistic way and discuss how you can start to make changes to this. By doing so, you can learn to see things in a more realistic light, which can help to reduce your anxiety levels. You might have unhelpful thoughts about all kinds of things. Here are some examples:

Being judged negatively by others:

- They think I'm useless

- They won't like me

Being unable to cope:

- I'll make a fool out of myself

- I'm too anxious to manage that

- I'll have a panic attack

Something terrible happening:

- What if I have an accident?

- What if I lose my job?

It is clear to see how this kind of thinking might make us anxious. Do you ever think in any of the ways outlined above?

You might find it difficult to identify an unhelpful thought. Try thinking about a time when you were feeling anxious. Consider what was running through your mind at that time.

Patterns of Unhelpful thinking

First, you need to be able to recognize an unhelpful thought. Then you can challenge it. Being aware of the common patterns that unhelpful thoughts follow can help you to recognize when you have them. Here are some of the common patterns that are unhelpful thoughts follow:

Predicting the Future:

When we are feeling anxious, it is common for us to spend a lot of time thinking about the future and predicting what could go wrong, rather than just letting things be. In the end, most of our predictions don't happen, and we have wasted time and energy being worried and upset about them.

For example:

- Assuming you will perform poorly at your job interview.

- Spending the week before an exam predicting you will fail, despite all your hard work studying and your previous good grades.

Mind Reading:

This means that you make assumptions about others' beliefs without having any real evidence to support them.

For example:

- My boss thinks I'm stupid

- People think I'm weird

Such ways of thinking naturally make us apprehensive.

Catastrophizing:

People commonly 'catastrophize' when they are anxious, which basically means that they often blow things out of proportion.

For example:

- They assume that something that has happened is far worse than it really is (e.g., that their friend is going to dislike them because they canceled a night out).

- They may think that something terrible is going to happen in the future when, in reality, there is very little evidence to support it (e.g., I'm going to get into serious trouble for calling in sick).

Focusing on the Negatives:

Anxious people often have a tendency to focus on the negatives, which keeps their anxiety going.

For example:

- They focus on the one person at work who doesn't like them, ignoring that they are very popular with the rest of their colleagues.

Should Statements:

People often imagine how they would like things to be or how they 'should be' rather than accepting how things really are.

For example:

- I should have got an A in History

- I should never be anxious

Unfortunately, when we do this, we are simply applying extra pressure to ourselves that can result in anxiety. Instead, it can sometimes help to accept that things can't always be perfect.

Over Generalizing:

Based on one isolated incident, you assume that all others will follow a similar pattern in the future.

For example:

- When enrolling in a college course, you meet a future classmate who you find irritating. As a result, you worry that everyone in the class will be the same and you won't make any friends.

"What If" Statements:

Have you wondered "what if" something bad happens?

For example:

- What if I have a panic attack at the party?

- What if I don't make friends when I start my new job?

This type of thought can make us avoid going places or doing things that we would like.

Labeling:

Do you find that you attach negative labels to yourself?

For example:

- I'm weak.

- I'm a waste of space.

- I'm always anxious.

Labels like this really influence how we see ourselves and can heighten our anxiety levels. Do any of your unhelpful thoughts follow some of these patterns? Create a two column list. On the left put down unhelpful thoughts and on the right add the category that corresponds. For example:

Unhelpful Thought	Category
"My boss thinks I'm useless"	Mind Reading
"My anxiety means I'm weak"	Labelling

We can learn techniques to challenge these unhelpful thoughts. This can help to reduce your anxiety levels. The next part of this handbook will discuss how we can go about challenging our unhelpful thoughts. You may come up with a more balanced thought that is accurate and based on evidence.

How to Challenge Unhelpful Thoughts

Once you have recognized an unhelpful thought, the next stage is to challenge it. To do this, you can ask yourself a series of questions. See the following example:

Situation: *The end of the year exams are approaching.*

How you feel: *Nervous, stressed, and apprehensive.*

Unhelpful thought: *I'll definitely fail my exams miserably!*

Challenges to an unhelpful thought

Now you can challenge your unhelpful thoughts by asking these questions.

Is there any evidence that contradicts these thoughts?

- I've always done well in my previous exams.

- I've been scoring well in my coursework.

Can you identify any of the patterns of unhelpful thinking described earlier?

- I'm 'predicting the future.' I have no evidence to suggest I'll fail.

What would you say to a friend who had this thought in a similar situation?

- I'd say don't be silly; you've always done well. As long as you've studied hard, you should be fine. Besides, you can only try your best.

What are the costs and benefits of thinking in this way?

- Costs: It's making me feel sick with worry.

- Benefits: I can't really think of any.

How will you feel about this in 6 months' time?

- I'll probably look back and laugh about how silly I was being.

Is there another way of looking at this situation?

- I've always done well in the past, so I should be OK. I can only do my best anyway; after all, I've studied hard. At worst, I'll just have to re-sit next year.

Once you have asked yourself these questions, you should read through your answers. Try to come up with a more balanced or rational view. For example:

Worrying about failing is doing me no good. I've always done well before, so I should be fine, especially since I've prepared properly.

Problem Solving

You might find it more difficult to cope if you have lots of problems that you can't seem to get on top of. This can have a clear impact on our anxiety levels. Struggling with unresolved problems can often make us feel worse. We can end up worrying or ruminating over our problems without finding a way to resolve them. This can make us feel even more upset and can end up interfering with our sleep.

It can help to develop a structured way of working through a problem. Beginning to overcome some of your problems might help you to feel better. You can improve your problem-solving skills by learning to apply the steps outlined here.

Identify your problem

The first thing to ask yourself is, "what's the problem?" Try to be as specific as possible.

For example:

- "I owe $400 to my friend."

- "I am going to miss this deadline."

Come up with possible solutions.

Try to list every way that you can think to overcome your problem. Don't worry about how unrealistic an idea seems. Write down anything and everything. The best solutions are likely to be the ones you think of yourself. This is because nobody really knows your situation as well as you do.

It may help to consider:

- How might you have solved similar problems in the past?

- What would your friend or family advise?

- How would you like to see yourself tackling the problem?

Choose a solution

Next, you need to select the best solution from your list. Think carefully about each option. It is useful to go through all the reasons 'for' and 'against' each idea. This will help you to make a good decision and select the best solution.

After this, you may find that you are still unsure. Perhaps a couple of approaches seem equally good. Try to pick one, to begin with. If it doesn't work, then you can always go back and try out a different one later.

Break down your solution

To help you carry out your chosen solution, it can be useful to break it down into smaller steps. This can make it easier and more manageable to follow through. The number of steps required will vary depending on the solution and how complex it is.

For example, someone with debt may have decided to try and resolve their problem by getting a part-time job. This would require several steps.

1. Buying a newspaper with job adverts

2. Choosing which job to apply for

3. Creating a resume

4. Sending out their resume

5. Buying Interview clothes

6. Preparing answers to potential interview questions

Try out your solution and review the outcome.

Follow the steps required to carry out your solution. Simply take them one at a time. Go at your own pace, and don't allow yourself to feel too rushed.

Once you have completed all the steps, you should then review the outcome. If you have successfully resolved your problem, then great. If the problem still exists, then don't give up.

- Is there another solution on your list that you could try?

- Is there a different solution that you have yet to consider?

- Can you ask someone else if they have any ideas or advice?

- Can you combine any of your solutions?

It is useful to remember that not all problems are within our control. This can make it really difficult, if not impossible, to resolve using the steps above. Perhaps you will have to wait or ask someone else to take action instead. In such a situation, try not to worry. *Nothing can be gained from worrying about something that you have no control over.*

Limiting the amount of time you spend worrying

Anxious people tend to spend much of their time worrying. Sometimes they worry to the point that they find it very hard to 'switch off' and relax. Indeed, one of the most frustrating things about feeling anxious is the seemingly uncontrollable worry that often occurs alongside it. Therefore, if we can reduce the amount of time we spend worrying, we can reduce our anxiety levels.

One way you can do this is to assign 'worry time.' This involves setting aside between fifteen and twenty minutes each day that you will allow yourself to worry. Any worries that pop into your head outside of 'worry time' should simply be noted and forgotten until later that day when you try to resolve them during your 'worry time.'

By noting them down, you can feel safe in the knowledge that you won't forget about attempting to resolve them later on. This should free up time during the day that is normally wasted worrying. Then - when your 'worry time' arrives, you should allow yourself to think about the things that have been worrying you that day and try to resolve them.

'Worry time' not only helps to reduce the time you spend worrying but also proves that you can have more control of whether you engage in worry or not. It also shows that worry is often unnecessary. This is because when you come back to consider your problems with a 'fresh eye,' many of them have often resolved themselves or simply seem less important.

See the steps below for more details:

1. Decide a time in the day that you will have your 'worry time.'

2. At other times, simply note down any worries that pop into your head and try to forget about them.

3. Once your 'worry time' arrives, choose how long you will allow yourself to 'worry' (try to keep it no longer than 15-20 minutes). Begin timing yourself so your 'worry time' doesn't overrun.

4. During worry time, try to resolve your worries proactively. Simply try to come up with solutions to your worries if possible. Using a pen and pad to jot down solutions can be helpful.

5. Stop as soon as your 'worry time' is finished. If any worries still feel unresolved, simply carry them over to tomorrow's 'worry time.'

Here are some handy hints to help you with your 'worry time.'

- If you find it difficult to switch off from all of your worries during the day, don't fret, as this should improve with time and practice.

- It may be useful to use the problem-solving section in this guide during 'worry time.'

- When it comes to 'worry time,' feel free to cut it short if you have resolved all of your worries early.

- Often things that have worried us at one point in the day seem less problematic when we re-visit them during 'worry time.' If this happens "great," simply forget about them.

- Remember, it is usually not possible to resolve every single worry or problem that you have. So if something is outside your control (or has already happened), try not to worry as you have done all you can. There is also the possibility that your worry won't even come true in the first place.

Relaxation

It is important to make time to relax and do activities that are enjoyable. This can help to reduce your anxiety levels by calming the body and mind. It can also help you to sleep. Without taking the time to unwind, it is easy to feel overwhelmed and stressed.

Relaxation can involve doing something that you enjoy or just being by yourself. Good examples might be reading a book or having a bath. Exercise is also particularly effective at helping us to relax. What you do does not really matter. Try to choose something that you will look forward to and that gives you a break. Doing an activity that you enjoy will also give you less time to spend worrying. Here is a list of activities that might help you to relax.

- Do some exercise (e.g. swim, cycle).

- Read a book.

- Watch your favorite TV show.

- Go to the cinema.

- Do something creative (e.g., draw, paint).

- Visit a friend or family member.

- Have a bath.

Try to add some of your own ideas into the box below or write them down on paper. You will know what works best for you.

Try to find time to relax every day. This might seem difficult, but it is worth making time for. It can help you to feel a lot better. There are audio relaxation guides available online that you might find helpful support. There are also some exercises described in the next few pages.

They are specifically designed to help you to relax. However, you should stop the exercise if at any time you begin to experience discomfort or pain.

Controlled breathing

This simple technique involves focusing on and slowing down our breathing patterns. Many people find this simple exercise very relaxing. It can be particularly helpful for those who feel dizzy or lightheaded when they feel worried or stressed. This sometimes happens because people's breathing changes and gets quicker when they feel distressed.

This can be an uncomfortable and unpleasant experience. It can make people even more on edge, and a vicious cycle can occur. Learning controlled breathing exercises can help you to manage these feelings more effectively. It can also help to give your mind and body a chance to calm down.

Remember, you can use this exercise to help you relax at any time. You could even use it to help you go to sleep. However, it is particularly useful if you ever feel lightheaded, dizzy, or faint.

Beginning: Get into a comfortable position. Ideally, sitting in an upright position with your feet firmly planted on the ground.

Middle: Work out a stable breathing rhythm. Perhaps try to breathe in for three seconds, hold this breath for two seconds, and then breathe out for three seconds. It can be helpful to count as you do this.

E.g. **IN: 1-2-3, HOLD: 1-2-3, OUT: 1-2-3, HOLD: 1-2-3, REPEAT.**

Ending: Repeat this action for a few minutes. You should soon begin to feel more relaxed. If you were feeling dizzy, then this should also get better after a few minutes.

Muscular relaxation

Tension often builds up when we feel upset or stressed. These symptoms can be painful and can cause anxiety in themselves. Muscular relaxation exercises can help you to control such unpleasant symptoms. They can reduce physical tension and help you to relax in general.

During this exercise, you have to tense and then relax different muscles in your body. You should focus on the feelings that you experience while doing this. With practice, you will then be more able to recognize and respond to the onset of tension.

You can work through as many muscle groups as you like. Don't feel that you have to cover every muscle in your whole body. It can be helpful to stick to the same muscle groups each time you practice. That way, you can get into a routine that you can easily remember. If you practice this nearly every day, you will probably notice an improvement after a couple of weeks.

Beginning: Find somewhere comfortable and quiet where you won't be interrupted. You can either sit or lie down to practice this exercise. Begin by focusing on your breathing. Try to have a slow and comfortable pace. You could use the controlled breathing technique described earlier. Do this for a few minutes to prepare for the muscular relaxation exercise.

Middle: Try to tense each muscle group for around five seconds. Don't tense the muscle too tight. Focus on the sensations that this brings. Then relax your muscles for a similar length of time, and again, focus on how this feels. Then move onto the next muscle group. Try to remember to keep your breathing at a comfortable pace throughout. Below are some suggestions of muscle groups that you may wish to work through:

- Legs - point your toes and tense your muscles as if you were trying to stand up.

- Stomach - tense your stomach muscles.

- Arms - make fists and tense your muscles as if you were trying to lift something.

- Shoulders - shrug your shoulders. Lift them up towards your ears.

- Face - make a frowning expression. Squeeze your eyes shut and screw up your nose.

Ending: It can be helpful to spend a few minutes just lying quietly in a relaxed state. See if you can notice any tension in your body and try to relax it. Otherwise, just let the tension be. If your mind wanders, try to bring your concentration back to your breathing. Finally, count down silently and slowly: **5 - 4 - 3 - 2 - 1 - 0**, and come out of the relaxation in your own time. See if it's possible to carry that relaxed feeling into whatever you do next.

Distraction

Distraction is a good technique to fend off symptoms of anxiety and stress when they feel overwhelming. This can also give you space to deal with a situation in a more considered and positive manner. It is also helpful when you don't have space or time to use a more proactive approach, such as a relaxation exercise.

Distraction simply involves trying to take your mind off uncomfortable symptoms or thoughts. You can do this by trying to focus on something unrelated. Often this helps them to pass.

Ideas to help distract you from your troubling thoughts or anxiety include:

- Try to appreciate small details in your surroundings.

- Count backward from 1000 in multiples of 7.

- Focus on your breathing, for example, the sensation of air as it flows in and out of your nose.

- Count things that you can see that begin with a particular letter.

- Visualize being in a pleasant, safe, and comfortable environment (e.g., being on a beach).

- Listen to your favorite music. Try to pick out all the different instruments and sounds that you can hear.

As with any relaxation exercise, it may take a few minutes before you begin to feel like it is working.

Reducing avoidance

People often get into the habit of avoiding situations that cause them difficulty. This coping strategy can, unfortunately, make the problem worse. This is because the longer we avoid something, the more intimidating it becomes. By avoiding situations, we also stop ourselves from proving that we can cope with them. As a result, our anxiety towards the situation continues, and our confidence remains low.

Take the example below:

Someone who tends to worry about being judged negatively by others.

Reaction:

- May avoid going out socially in case people don't like them or they make a fool of themselves. For instance, they may avoid going to work nights out, parties, restaurants, or taking part in a hobby.

- May avoid speaking when in large groups, instead of staying quiet and not really 'being themselves.'

- May avoid all performance situations, such as giving a speech or showing off a piece of work, due to their fear of being negatively evaluated.

Outcome:

By avoiding all of these related situations, they never have a chance to practice in them or prove that they could cope well.

It is easy to see how using avoidance as a strategy to cope can soon begin to have a negative impact on people's lives as they start to avoid more and more situations.

If, instead, we confront difficult situations, then it is possible to build up our confidence. This will help your anxiety to reduce significantly.

List the things that you avoid.

Come up with a list of the situations that you often try to escape from or avoid.

For example:

Things I Avoid	Predicted anxiety
Going on a work night out	
Speaking in front of small groups	
Going out for a meal with friends	
Submitting new ideas to my boss	
Joining a yoga class	
Speaking in front of a large group of friends	
Delivering formal presentations at work	

Ranking these situations

Rank your list of situations in order of difficulty. From the least anxiety-provoking to the most anxiety-provoking on a scale of 0 -10. 0 = no anxiety and 10 = extreme anxiety.

For examples:

Things I Avoid	Predicted anxiety
Going on a work night out	6
Speaking in front of small groups	5
Going out for a meal with friends	2
Submitting new ideas to my boss	3
Joining a yoga class	9
Speaking in front of a large group of friends	8
Delivering formal presentations at work	7

Once you have done this, try to organize your items from least anxiety-provoking to most anxiety-provoking.

Confronting the lowest-ranked situation

Try to confront the lowest-ranked item on your list. This will be the item that causes you the least anxiety. You will likely find that although your anxiety might initially rise, it will drop if you remain in the situation for long enough. Try to stay with the situation until your anxiety has reduced by at least half.

Repeating this task

Repeat the task as often as possible (every day if you can). Try not to leave too long between times when you confront this item. This is because the more you confront something, the more your fear will reduce. You should notice your anxiety getting less and less each time you do so. You may find eventually that it will cause you little or no anxiety at all.

Moving on to the next lowest item

When you feel comfortable with an item, try to move on to the next item on your list. Working through your list, you will begin to feel anxious in fewer and fewer situations. You should find that your confidence grows as you move on from each item. You should find that tasks ranked as more difficult seem more manageable as you progress.

Things to consider:

- Don't fear the symptoms of anxiety. Anxiety is a natural and healthy reaction that is not dangerous.

- Try not to escape situations you fear half-way through. Stay, and your anxiety will eventually decrease.

- Your anxiety will reduce each time you confront a feared situation. Try to confront your fears as often as possible.

- You may also find it helpful to challenge any unhelpful thoughts as you face a fear.

- Look out for other situations that you avoid due to anxiety. Try to gradually reduce your avoidance more and more.

- You may confront an item on your list which doesn't go as well as you had hoped. Try not to give up. Persevere, and it should eventually get easier.

- If an item on your list seems too hard, see if you can put in an extra step or two before it. This will allow your confidence to rise further before you face it.

Nothing can be gained from worrying about something that you have no control over.

Part 2: Depression

Depression is classified as a mood disorder. It may be described as feelings of sadness, loss, or anger that interfere with a person's everyday activities. Depression is a mood disorder that involves a persistent feeling of sadness and loss of interest. It is different from the mood fluctuations that people regularly experience as a part of life.

Depression is an ongoing problem, not a passing one. It consists of episodes during which the symptoms last for at least two weeks. Depression can last for several weeks, months, or years.

People experience depression in different ways. It may interfere with your daily work, resulting in lost time and lower productivity. It can also influence relationships and some chronic health conditions.

Depression most often results from a combination of factors rather than one single cause. For example, if you went through a divorce, were diagnosed with a serious medical condition, or lost your job, the stress could prompt you to start drinking more, which in turn could cause you to withdraw from family and friends. Those factors combined could then trigger depression.

The following are examples of risk factors that can make you more susceptible to developing depression:

Loneliness and isolation: Thers'e a strong relationship between loneliness and depression. Not only can lack of social support heighten your risk for depression but having depression can cause you to withdraw from others, exacerbating feelings of isolation. Having anyone to talk to, especially close friends or family can help you maintain perspective on your issues and avoid dealing with problems alone.

Marital or relationship problems: While a network of strong and supportive relationships can be crucial to good mental health, troubled, unhappy, or abusive

- obesity

It's important to realize that feeling down at times is a normal part of life. Sad and upsetting events happen to everyone. But, if you're feeling down or hopeless regularly, you could be dealing with depression.

Depression differs from simple grief or mourning, which are appropriate emotional responses to the loss of loved persons or objects. There are clear grounds for a person's unhappiness; depression is considered present if the depressed mood is disproportionately long or severe vis-à-vis the precipitating event.

The distinctions between the duration of depression, the circumstances under which it arises, and certain other characteristics underlie the classification of depression into different types. Examples of different types of depression include bipolar disorder, major depressive disorder (clinical depression), persistent depressive disorder, and seasonal affective disorder.

Diagnosing Depression

Depression is mainly diagnosed by history and clinical examinations, or a specific pattern of symptoms. Still, if you have symptoms like sleep or appetite changes, your doctor may look into other conditions unrelated to mental health (a thyroid issue is a classic example).

Treatments for Depression

There are ever-evolving ways to treat depression, and which mix will work for you will depend on everything from how long you've had it and the severity of your symptoms.

Medications

There's no shame in taking medication to manage your depression. People routinely take medication for physical ailments, and having a mental illness isn't any different.

If you're worried about the possible side effects, remember that any medication can be tapered down or ceased.

Therapy

Who doesn't go to therapy these days? It's as much a part of the regular conversation as the weather. Psychotherapy (aka talk therapy), sometimes along with medication, can be highly beneficial in treating, managing, and reducing the duration of an episode of depression.

"Evidence-based treatments, such as Cognitive Behavioral Therapy (CBT), Acceptance and Commitment Therapy, and Dialectical Behavior Therapy, are very effective in treating depression. "These psychotherapies are active skills-based therapies that help individuals develop and maintain skills to manage difficult thoughts and feelings."

Trained experts like psychiatrists and psychologists can offer many types of these treatments, from light therapy for seasonal affective disorder to CBT, to change your thought processes. One goal of CBT includes behavioral activation, effective treatment and technique in which a therapist can help you schedule more enjoyable activities that bring fulfillment, meaning, or pleasure into your life.

Healthy Habits

Incorporating new healthy habits is a useful way to combat depression. Meditation is one highly effective way of clearing your head and calming your body. You can also try keeping a journal—some people find that it helps express their thoughts on paper instead of bottling them inside. Talk to close friends and family about your struggles, too. Having a social support system plays a key part in maintaining your mental health and wellbeing.

Recovery is a journey, not a destination. Bad days will still come, but with well-targeted treatment, you should overcome extreme lows. While science has yet to find a cure for mental disorders such as depression, it is entirely possible to live a happy and fulfilling life despite it.

Depression and Suicide Risk

Depression usually does not lead to suicide ideation. Studies have shown that about two percent of people treated for depression in an outpatient setting will die by suicide. If the treatment is inpatient, the number doubles to four percent. Men are more likely to die by suicide after depression than women.

Depression and Diet

What foods help ease depression? While no specific diet has been proven to relieve depression, a healthy diet can help you feel your best physically and mentally. Certain foods may be linked to brain health and support for memory, alertness, and mood. Examples include foods that contain omega-3 fatty acids (found in nuts and fatty fish like salmon), antioxidants (blueberries, broccoli), and nutrients like choline (found in egg yolk). Always talk

with your doctor before making any major diet changes.

Depression and Brain Chemicals

It's often said that depression results from a chemical imbalance, but that speech does not capture how complex it is. Research suggests that depression doesn't spring from simply having too much or too little of certain brain chemicals. Rather, there are many possible causes of depression, including faulty mood regulation by the brain, genetic vulnerability, stressful life events, medications, and medical problems. It's believed that several of these forces interact to bring on depression.

To be sure, chemicals are involved in this process, but it is not a simple matter of one chemical being too low and another too high. Rather, many chemicals are involved, working both inside and outside nerve cells. There are millions, even billions, of chemical reactions that make up the dynamic system responsible for your mood, perceptions, and life experience.

With this complexity level, you can see how two people might have similar depression symptoms. Still, what treatments will work best, may be entirely different.

Researchers have learned much about the biology of depression. They've identified genes that make individuals more vulnerable to low moods and influence how they respond to drug therapy. One day, these discoveries should lead to better, more individualized treatment (see "From the lab to your medicine cabinet"). And while researchers know more now than ever before about how the brain regulates mood, their understanding of the biology of depression is far from complete.

What follows is an overview of the current understanding of the major factors believed to play a role in the causes of depression.

The brain's impact on depression

Popular lore has it that emotions reside in the heart. Science, though, tracks the seat of your emotions to the brain. Certain areas of the brain help regulate mood. Researchers believe that — more important than levels of specific brain chemicals — nerve cell connections, nerve cell growth, and nerve circuits' functioning have a major impact on depression. Still, their understanding of the neurological underpinnings of mood is incomplete.

Typically, the **symptoms associated with depression** are the same, although the number and intensity would be unique to each person. The following are the most commonly seen.

- Change in sleep
- Reduced or increased appetite
- Concentration difficulty
- Loss of interest in normal activities
- Sad mood
- Feelings of worthlessness or guilt

- Loss of energy (Fatigue)
- Suicidal thoughts

If you are experiencing any one or a combination of these symptoms, you need to learn ways of dealing with depression. Unfortunately, some people will have all of these symptoms but remain in denial that anything is wrong. Instead, they will go about life moping, crying, and feeling defeated, and often unsuccessful in business and relationships. This is not living but merely existing. Instead of allowing this disease to ruin or control your life, learn strategies for dealing with depression that will allow you to enjoy life again.

In most cases, some type of intervention is needed. This may involve talking to a counselor or going on antidepressant medication, which is nothing to be embarrassed or ashamed of. Seeking help shows that you are a responsible individual interested in getting better. Keep in mind; doctors may need to try several treatment options before finding the one that works best for the type of depression you have, so remain patient.

Dealing with depression also means realizing that this is a serious health/mental disease. The good news is that when treated quickly and appropriately, people do get better, going on to live happy and productive lives. However, individuals who refuse to see depression for what it is are more likely to struggle and be miserable. Being realistic will also allow you to examine the reasons for the depression, which, once identified, can be corrected.

For example, you might be feeling depressed because the kids have all moved out of the house. Now, as a single adult, you feel isolated, alone, and even abandoned. Understanding the underlying cause of the depression can provide you with hope for dealing with the depression. With this, you can begin to build a new life, one focused around other single adults and activities. You could redecorate the home, changing things to your preference that are not so kid-orientated. Remain positive, knowing that understanding and dealing with depression provides an opportunity for a new lease on life.

Most importantly, never feel as if you have been singled out. Millions of people suffer from depression right along with you, so you are certainly not being picked on, nor are you alone. However, with any depression, gaining control over it will make all the difference in the work.

If you want to know how to deal with depression, you need some practical advice to help you climb out of this hellish state of mind forever. Life is a privilege, and to live it fully and make your unique contribution to the world, you only need to follow some simple steps.

One important way of dealing with depression is to **eat right**. Fresh, natural foods, especially colorful vegetables. Energy creates motivation, and motivation allows you to make the changes that will help you create a brand new life. Focus on drinking lots of water, eating fresh vegetables in season and eating lean protein from meat, fish, nuts or legumes at every meal.

Another important answer to how to deal with depression is to get some form of **daily exercise**. Exercise does not have to be strenuous. Instead, focus on making it fun. Do something that invigorates you and leaves you feeling better. Walking the dog is exercise. Riding your bike around the neighborhood is another form of exercise that you might enjoy. Focus on the joy of movement. You can even jump on a mini-trampoline while you watch your favorite TV show. There are so many choices today. Mix things up to prevent boredom and to keep discovering new activities.

Severity of depression

The severity of depression can vary from person to person. Severity is generally based on the number of symptoms you have from the list of symptoms. The list of symptoms again:

- Change in sleep
- Reduced or increased appetite
- Concentration difficulty
- Loss of interest in normal activities
- Sad mood
- Feelings of worthlessness or guilt
- Loss of energy (Fatigue)
- Suicidal thoughts

Severity is categorized as follows:

Severe depression - you would normally have most or all of the eight symptoms listed above. Also, symptoms markedly interfere with your normal functioning.

Moderate depression - you would normally have more than five symptoms needed to make the diagnosis of depression. Also, symptoms will usually include both core symptoms. Also, the severity of symptoms or impairment of your functioning is between mild and severe.

Mild depression - you would normally have five of the symptoms listed above required to make the diagnosis of depression. However, you are not likely to have more than five or six of the symptoms. Also, your normal functioning is only mildly impaired.

Subthreshold depression - you have fewer than the five symptoms needed to make a diagnosis of depression. So, it is not classed as depression. But, the symptoms you do have are troublesome and cause distress. If this situation persists for more than two years, it is sometimes called dysthymia.

What causes depression?

The exact cause is not known. Anyone can develop depression. Some people are more prone to it, and it can develop for no apparent reason. You may have no particular problem or worry, but symptoms can develop quite suddenly. So, there may be some genetic factor involved that makes some people more prone than others to depression. 'Genetic' meanig that the condition is passed on through families.

An episode of depression may also be triggered by a life event such as a relationship problem, bereavement, redundancy, illness, etc. In many people, it is a mixture of the two. For example, the combination of a mild low mood with some life problems, such as work stress, may lead to a spiral down into depression.

Women tend to develop depression more often than men. Particularly common times for women to become depressed are after childbirth.

Symptoms and Diagnosis

Symptoms of depression vary widely but can be divided into three main categories:

- **Emotional and cognitive (thinking) symptoms**: This include a depressed mood, lack of interest or motivation in things you typically enjoy, problems making decisions, irritability, excessive worrying, memory problems and excessive guilt.

- **Physical symptoms**: This includes fatigue, sleep problems (such as waking too early, problems falling or staying asleep, sleeping too much), appetite changes, weight loss or gain, aches and pains, headaches, and burning or tingling sensations.

- **Behavioral symptoms:** This includes crying uncontrollably, having angry outbursts, withdrawing from friends and family, becoming a workaholic, abusing alcohol or drugs, cutting or otherwise hurting yourself, and, in the worst cases, considering or attempting suicide.

How To Deal With Depression

In some ways, the period between ages 18 and 29 is the best. It's that time when you get to develop a sense of independence in college, start new jobs, scout out the dating scene, or head off to new cities.

On the other hand, it's a time often characterized by debt, romantic misadventures, loneliness, and a sense of uncertainty about who you are and why you're here.

It's not surprising that people in their late teens and their 20s are especially vulnerable to depression.

Symptoms of depression in early age

The symptoms of depression can range from subtle to super severe. It's important to talk to a doctor or therapist you trust rather than a DIY diagnosis. That said, here are some of the common symptoms that can clue you in:

- **Behaviors**: You're not interested in things you used to love. You feel tired a lot. Maybe you think about death and suicide sometimes. You're drinking more alcohol or using drugs.

- **Cognition**: You have trouble concentrating or completing tasks on your to-do list. In conversation, it takes you longer to respond than it used to. You feel like it's tougher to make decisions.

- **Emotions**: When you think about life, things feel kind of pointless. You may feel empty, sad, hopeless, indifferent, or guilty.

- **Mood**: Things have started to set you off more easily, or maybe you're irritated and anxious about things that didn't bother you before.

- **Physical symptoms**: Your body has aches and pains, or maybe you get unexplained headaches. Maybe you're losing weight because food is kind of "meh" right now. The opposite can happen too — maybe you're turning to comfort foods way more than usual.

- **Psychomotor**: You feel like you can't sit still. You feel agitated and restless, or maybe you pace around the room.

- **Sex**: You're not as interested in sex as you used to be.

- **Sleep:** You're sleeping a lot more and at different hours than you used to. Or maybe you have trouble falling asleep or staying asleep, and it's hard to get back to sleep if you wake up in the middle of the night.

Causes for young adult

Today's 20-somethings are going through several psychosocial and biological experiences that make them especially vulnerable to depression.

For one thing, depression is often triggered by loss; the period between ages 18 and 29 is filled with potential losses:

Breaking up: with a significant other, losing friends, losing a job, failing in school or not getting into an academic program, or realizing that your dream career plans might not work out.

Biological factors

Biological factors also come into play. In the last decade, scientists have found that the frontal lobe (the part of your brain responsible for planning and reasoning) doesn't completely develop until the mid-20s.

This means 20-somethings are faced with making some huge decisions (where to live, what career to pursue, whether to propose) when they aren't yet at their full cognitive capacity, causing feelings of angst and anxiety.

Consumption of Alcohol

In some cases, 20-somethings might not realize certain lifestyle factors can contribute to depressive symptoms, like alcohol, which acts as a depressant.

The good news is that these emotions are pretty common and typically pass when people hit 30. But depression can still be a serious issue that often requires some kind of treatment. Here's how to address those feelings when they pop up.

Managing depression – Self-help tips

No matter what point someone is at in their depression and recovery, they can do things to take care of themselves. That means taking care of both the body and the mind. Here are some self-help tips you can share:

- Eat right, sleep right, get outside, move your body! All of these basic healthy behaviors can make a positive difference to your whole body-mind system.

- Avoid alcohol and street drugs. These may seem like a way to make you feel better, but they can make things a lot worse and prevent recovery in the long run.

- Find ways to reduce stress where and when you can. Try out yoga or tai chi, or learn how to meditate.

- Keep a journal of your thoughts and feelings. Try to come up with one or two things you're grateful for every day and make a note of them.

- Express yourself creatively. For example, dance, draw or make music.

Mindfulness and Meditation Styles

It's estimated that 95% of our behavior runs on autopilot. Thats' because neural networks underlie all of our habits, reducing our millions of sensory inputs per second into manageable shortcuts so we can function in this crazy world. These default brain signals are so efficient that they often cause us to relapse into old behaviors before we remember what we meant to do instead.

Mindfulness is the exact opposite of these default processes. It's executive control rather than autopilot, and enables intentional actions, willpower, and decisions. But that takes practice. The more we activate the intentional brain, the stronger it gets. Every time we do something deliberate and new, we stimulate neuroplasticity, activating our grey matter, which is full of newly sprouted neurons that have not yet been groomed for autopilot brain.

But hers'e the problem: While our intentional brain knows what is best for us, our autopilot brain causes us to shortcut our way through life. So how can we trigger ourselves to be mindful when we need it most? This is where the notion of "behavior design" comes in. It's a way to put your intentional brain in the driver's seat. There are two ways to do that—first, slowing down the autopilot brain by putting obstacles in its way, and second, removing obstacles in the path of the intentional brain, so it can gain control.

Shifting the balance to give your intentional brain more power takes some work, though. Here are some ways to get started:

- Put meditation reminders around you. If you intend to do some yoga or to meditate, put your yoga mat or your meditation cushion in the middle of your floor so you can't miss it as you walk by.

- Refresh your reminders regularly. Say you decide to use sticky notes to remind yourself of a new intention. That might work for about a week, but then your autopilot brain and old habits take over again. Try writing new notes to yourself; add variety or make them funny. That way they'll stick with you longer.

- Create new patterns. You could try a series of "If this, then that" messages to create easy reminders to shift into the intentional brain. For instance, you might come up with, "If office door, then deep breath," as a way to shift into mindfulness as you are about to start your workday. Or, "If phone rings, take a breath before answering." Each intentional action to shift into mindfulness will strengthen your intentional brain.

Introduction to Basic Breathing Meditation.

The easiest way to begin meditation is to focus deliberately on your breathing, while letting go of distractions as they come up. One technique used by Buddhist practitioners is to sit in an upright position, and breath in and out of your nose while focusing on the sensation of the air flowing through your nostrils, with as little physical effort as possible. Repeat this gentle breathing and try to only focus on the sensation of the air flowing in order to clear your mind from other distractions. This takes time and repetition, so don't get discouraged. Keep bringing your attention back to your breathing.

Some other helpful breathing meditation techniques to remove distraction that can also be used include:

- Focusing on the rise and fall of your chest.
- Repeating a mantra (e.g. I am me.)
- Notice and relax tense parts of your body
- Touch forefingers and thumb for added help with focus

More Styles of Mindfulness Meditation

Once you have explored a basic seated meditation practice, you might want to consider other forms of meditation including walking and lying down. Whereas the previous meditations used the breath as a focal point for practice, these meditations below focus on different parts of the body.

Introduction to the Body Scan Meditation.

Try this: Sit in an upright position with your feet touching the ground. Feel your feet on the ground. In your shoes or without, it doesn't matter. Then track or scan over your whole body, bit by bit—slowly

—all the way up to the crown of your head. The point of this practice is to check in with your whole body: Fingertips to shoulders, butt to big toe. Only rules are: No judging, no wondering, no worrying (all activities your mind may want to do); just check in with the physical feeling of being in your body. Aches and pains are fine. You don't have to do anything about anything here. You're just noticing. Begin to focus your attention on different parts of your body. You can spotlight one particular area or go through a sequence like this: toes, feet (sole, heel, top of foot), through the legs, pelvis, abdomen, lower back, upper back, chest, arms down to the fingers, shoulders, neck, different parts of the face, and head. For each part of the body, linger for a few moments and notice the different sensations as you focus.

The moment you notice that your mind has wandered, return your attention to the part of the body you last remember.

If you fall asleep during this body-scan practice, that's okay. When you realize you've been nodding off, take a deep breath to help you reawaken and perhaps reposition your body (which will also help wake it up). When you're ready, return your attention to the part of the body you last remember focusing on.

Introduction to the Walking Meditation

Fact: Most of us live pretty sedentary lives, leaving us to build extra-curricular physical activity into our days to counteract all that. Point is: Mindfulness doesn't have to feel like another thing on your to-do list. It can be injected into some of the activities you're already doing. Hers'e how to integrate a mindful walking practice into your day.

As you begin, walk at a natural pace. Place your hands wherever comfortable: on your belly, behind your back, or at your sides:

- If you find it useful, you can count steps up to 10, and then start back at one again. If you're in a small space, as you reach ten, pause, and with intention, choose a moment to turn around.

- With each step, pay attention to the lifting and falling of your foot. Notice movement in your legs and the rest of your body. Notice any shifting of your body from side to side.

- Whatever else captures your attention, come back to the sensation of walking. Your mind will wander, so without frustration, guide it back again as many times as you need.

- Particularly outdoors, maintain a larger sense of the environment around you, taking it all in, staying safe and aware.

Introduction to Loving-Kindness Meditation

You cannot will yourself into particular feelings toward yourself or anyone else. Rather, you can practice reminding yourself that you deserve happiness and ease and that the same goes for your child, your family, your friends, your neighbors, and everyone else in the world. This loving-kindness practice involves silently repeating phrases that offer good qualities to oneself and to others.

1. You can start by taking delight in your own goodness—calling to mind things you have done out of good-heartedness, and rejoicing in those memories to celebrate the potential for goodness we all share.

2. Silently recite phrases that reflect what we wish most deeply for ourselves in an enduring way. Traditional phrases are:

- May I live in safety.

- May I have mental happiness (peace, joy).

- May I have physical happiness (health, freedom from pain).

- May I live with ease.

3. Repeat the phrases with enough space and silence between so they fall into a rhythm that is pleasing to you. Direct your attention to one phrase at a time.

4. Each time you notice your attention has wandered, *be kind to yourself* and let go of the distraction. Come back to repeating the phrases without judging or disparaging yourself.

5. After some time, visualize yourself in the center of a circle composed of those who have been kind to you, or have inspired you because of their love. Perhaps you've met them, or read about them; perhaps they live now, or have existed historically or even mythically. That is the circle. As you visualize yourself in the center of it, experience yourself as the recipient of their love and attention. Keep gently repeating the phrases of loving-kindness for yourself.

6. To close the session, let go of the visualization, and simply keep repeating the phrases for a few more minutes. Each time you do so, you are transforming your old, hurtful relationship to yourself, and are moving forward, sustained by the force of kindness.

FAQ on Mindfulness Meditation

When you're new to meditation, its' natural for questions to pop up often. These answers may ease your mind.

1) If I have an itch, can I scratch it?

Yes—however, first try scratching it with your mind before using your fingers.

2) Should I breathe fast or slow or in between?

Only worry if you've stopped breathing. Otherwise, you're doing fine. Breathe in whatever way feels comfortable to you.

3) Should my eyes be open or closed?

No hard-and-fast rules. Try both. If open, not too wide, and with a soft, slightly downward gaze, not focusing on anything in particular. If closed, not too hard, and not imagining anything in particular in your mind's eye.

4) Is it possible I'm someone who just CANNOT meditate?

When you find yourself asking that question, your meditation has officially begun. Everyone wonders that. Notice it. Escort your attention back to your object of focus (the breath). When you're lost and questioning again, come back to the breathe again. Thats' the practice. There's no limit to the number of times you can be distracted and come back to the breath. Meditating is not a race to perfection—*Its' returning again and again to the breath.*

5) Is it better to practice in a group or by myself?

Both are great! It's enormously supportive to meditate with others. And, practicing on your own builds discipline.

6) Whats' the best time of day to meditate? Whatever works. Consider your circumstances: children, pets, work. Experiment. But watch out. If you always choose the most convenient time, it will usually be tomorrow.

7) Do you have any tips on integrating pets into meditation practice?

While meditating, we don't have to fight off distractions like a knight slaying dragons. If your dog or cat comes into the room and barks and meows and brushes up against you or settles down on a part of your cushion, no big deal. Let it be. What works less well is to interrupt your session to relate to them. If thats' whats' going to happen, try to find a way to avoid their interrupting your practice.

How Much Should I Meditate?

Meditation is no more complicated than what w'eve described above. It is that simple ... and that challenging. It's also powerful and worth it. The key is to commit to sit every day, even if it's for five minutes. Meditation teacher Sharon Salzberg says: "One of my meditation teachers said that the most important moment in your meditation practice is the moment you sit down to do it. Because right then you're saying to yourself that you believe in change, you believe in caring for yourself, and you're making it real. You're not just holding some value like mindfulness or compassion in the abstract, but really making it real."

Now that you have an introduction to the world of meditation, and see how varied it can be, try to find which style work best for you. Do more research and look into different meditation techniques. You can try to search for a "meditation guide" online for a more in depth look at specific meditation styles.

Music and the Perception of Anxiety

Music can have an overwhelming effect on our moods. Just think of the way you feel when that pop song from when you were a child comes on the radio (or streaming service). You instantly get flooded with old emotions, memories, and sensations.

In more than one way, the effect of music on your mood can be used as a tool to help with depression and anxiety. Certain types of music can have specific effects on our mood. Loud, thumping music can get us into a hyped up mood whereas soft, serene tones can lull us into relaxation. So, whether you're trying to put yourself in the right mindset for meditation or your next dentist's visit, calming music can help aid in preparing your mind and mood.

Dental care is considered one of the five most commonly feared situations and one of the main reasons for missing dental appointments. Music therapy has been used as a non-pharmacological method to control anxiety due to its suppressive action on the sympathetic nervous system, leading to a reduction in both adrenaline production and neuromuscular activation, thus reducing the patient's anxiety.

In dentistry, the use of music has proven to reduce the physiological parameters of anxiety in patients during dental cleaning, extractions, endodontic treatments, and pediatric care. One of the most objective and simple ways to measure stress and anxiety is through salivary cortisol. Studies have shown that music significantly reduces saliva cortisol levels during simulated dental care situations, such as showing the patient the carpule syringe needle and exposure to a high-speed dental hand piece sound. In this regard, it has been described that music is effective in controlling anxiety.

Considering that the measurement of salivary cortisol allows to identify the stress levels of patients undergoing dental extractions, this study aimed to evaluate the effect of music at 432 Hz and

440 Hz, versus no music, on anxiety levels according to the CORAH Modified Dental Anxiety Scale (CORAH-MDAS), and the salivary cortisol levels of patients requiring a simple dental extraction.

432 Hz Frequency Sounds

Sound frequencies are thought by some to have specific effects on the body, but for purposes of mindfulness we can use them to create an environment of calmness. But which frequencies are most peaceful? According to the International Organization for Standardization (ISO), the pitch standard established for the musical note A is 440 Hz. However, it has been noted that the tones of the 440 Hz tuning frequency can be uncomfortable, irritating and disagreeable, whereas the intervals and tones obtained from the *432 Hz* tuning frequency are peaceful, pleasant and more harmonious.

Anxiety caused by dental treatment is a complex issue conditioned by personality characteristics, fear of pain, past traumatic dental experiences particularly in childhood, or the influence of anxious relatives, which manifests as increased anxiety and salivary cortisol levels before tooth extractions. However, music has proved to be effective in anxiety control. Di Nasso, et al. 11 (2016) studied the impact of music at 432 Hz in patients undergoing endodontic (root canal) treatment, showing that blood pressure and heart rate decreased significantly compared to a control group, suggesting that music affects the autonomic nervous system, and the patient's musical preference could have a greater positive impact than the operators'.

The explanation for the effect of music tuned at 432 Hz for anxiety control could rely on the spectral centroid theory, which postulates that the musical note A=432 Hz contains different or superior sound qualities, and details how the perception of a sound can be drastically modified when the frequency spectrum changes.

Still, Di Nasso's study showed that music at both 432 Hz and 440 Hz significantly reduced clinical anxiety levels according to the CORAH-MDAS compared to the control group; and that emotional response and perception of anxiety when using the CORAH-MDAS do not show significant differences between musical frequencies (432 Hz – 440 Hz). Therefore, the reduction in clinical stress awareness is probably linked to the listener's interpretations, his or her associations, and mental constructions, rather than to any innate pitch attribute.

However, regarding the physiological parameter of salivary cortisol, they observed that music at 432 Hz had significantly smaller concentrations than the control group. They found similar results on plasma cortisol levels during and three postoperative hours in patients undergoing general surgery, suggesting a physiological explanation because nitric oxide may be responsible for reducing anxiety and stress in response to music therapy, probably as part of a complex interrelationship between emotional centers within the central nervous system.

On the other hand, a report by Stefano, et al.(2004) showed that there was a statistically significant increase in opiate receptors in mononuclear cells in subjects undergoing pre and post-musical intervention, finding that IL-6 levels were significantly lower in peripheral blood plasma samples compared to the control group.

The authors define the type of music applied in musical medicine studies as "relaxing", such as classical music or music described as "calming for the patient," the melodies of pianos and guitars, latin chant and non-musical acoustic control (e.g., sound of waves), which allow a standardization in the effect of anxiety control.

A meta-analysis by Pelletier (2004) concludes that musical stimuli selected arbitrarily have a more significant effect on stress reduction than music chosen by the patients themselves, because they might be associated with an event that induces a previously conceived emotion.

Therefore, it stimulates the patient rather than increase relaxation. Moreover, according to the effect of music on physiological responses a study by Bradt, et al. (2013) suggests that listening to music has a small impact on heart rate variability, blood pressure and respiratory frequency, but more research on this topic is needed.

Comparing music intervention at different frequencies is somewhat controversial, mainly because no other study provides a precedent that different frequencies of the same musical composition are more pleasant or harmonious. Despite these limitations, these studies show the levels of anxiety and salivary cortisol before and after musical intervention at different frequencies, being the first report in this area to determine the effectiveness of music therapy at varying frequencies to control dental treatment anxiety.

Although still controversial, sounds and music in particular, have been proven to have an effect on our mood. For use with meditation and mindfulness, harmonious music can help tame your overthinking and create a sense of calm that will enhance the meditation experience. Search online for 432 Hz music and try it out for yourself.

Meditation Music - 432 Hz on YouTube

Search *"432 Hz Music"* on YouTube: https://www.youtube.com/results?search_query=432hz+music

Conclusion

Anxiety and depression are common and becoming more so. Understanding what these two conditions are is the first step in dealing with them. Hopefully this handbook has been able to give you a better understanding of what anxiety and depression entail and offered practical ways to deal with them in your daily life.

Whether you're combatting negative thinking or working on getting over a deeply held fear, there are tools and techniques throughout this handbook to help you along the way.

Again, utilize this handbook as a way to traverse the often uncomfortable feelings and behaviors that come with anxiety and depression. Whenever you need to, go back to the start and work through each section at your own pace. Give yourself time and be patient.

... and remember:

Nothing can be gained from worrying about something that you have no control over.

****If you ever get thoughts of harming yourself, tell someone you trust or if you feel like you have no one to talk to, reach out to a help line. You are never alone.****

Crisis Hotline Resources

- <u>National Suicide Prevention Hotline</u> -- 1-800-273-8255

- <u>Crisis Text Line</u> -- Text Hello to 741741

- <u>YouthLine</u> -- Text teen2teen to 839863, or call 1-877-968-8491

If you found this handbook helpful, please leave an honest review.